Introduction

Life, in all its complexity, often presents us with unanticipated guests—those fleeting moments that arrive without warning, shifting our perception of the world. For some, these guests come in the form of joy, love, or epiphanies. But for others, these visitors are darker, more sinister, challenging the very fabric of their existence. For Rose, her uninvited guest came not in the form of a person or an event, but as a force—an inevitable truth that she had spent her entire life avoiding: Death.

This is a story about fear, transformation, and the ancient wisdom that offered Rose a way to transcend her deepest terror. It is not just the tale of one woman but a reminder that every breath we take can be a bridge between fear and peace.

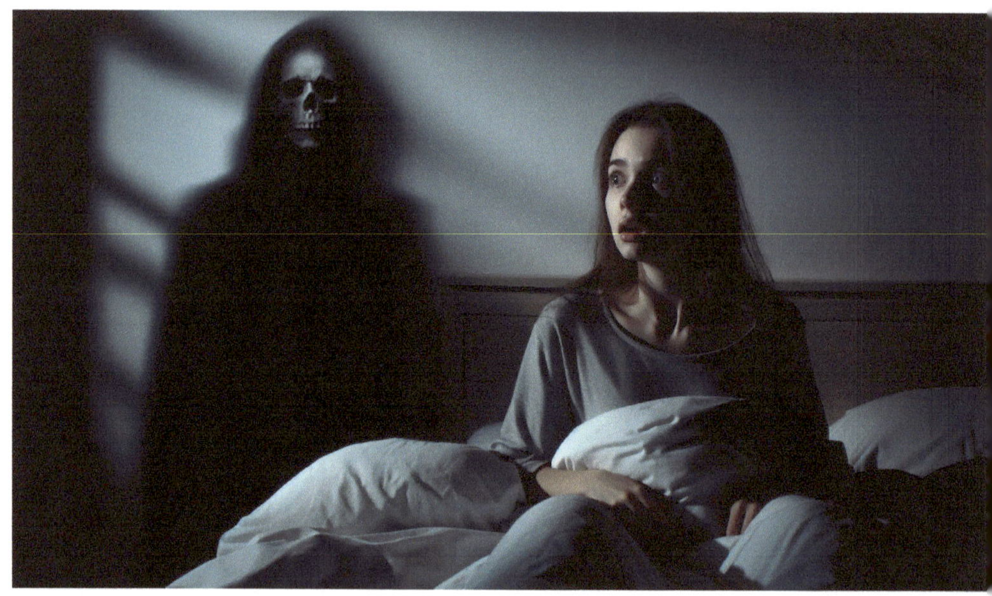

The Midnight Visitor

Rose sat in her dimly lit apartment, the hum of the city just outside her window barely registering in her mind. The day had been exhausting— endless meetings, deadlines, and small talk that felt more draining than any physical exertion. She rubbed her temples, trying to will away the growing tension.

The clock on the wall struck midnight, its soft chimes echoing through the quiet room. As she reached for her cup of tea, a cold draft swept across the room, chilling her skin. She frowned, her eyes darting towards the window. It was closed.

Strange.

She shrugged it off, but an uneasy feeling settled in her chest. As she rose to head toward the bedroom, she saw it—a shadow. A tall, dark figure, standing still by the doorway. Rose froze, her heart pounding in her chest.

Who could it be? How did they get in?

Her mind raced with possibilities, none of which made sense. The figure didn't move. It simply stood there, an outline against the darkness. It wasn't threatening, nor did it feel particularly human. She blinked, trying to convince herself it was a trick of the light, a product of her overworked mind. But the shadow remained.

"Who are you?" she whispered, her voice shaky.

The figure stepped forward, but there was no sound—no creak of the floor, no footsteps. Rose's breath caught in her throat. The closer it came, the more distinct it became. Tall, cloaked in black, with a face that wasn't a face at all, but a void—a darkness deeper than the night.

"Rose," it whispered, in a voice that was both soft and chilling. She gasped, stepping backward, her body trembling with fear. How did this thing know her name?

"Wh-what do you want?" she stammered, clutching the edge of the sofa, her knuckles turning white.

The figure didn't respond. It only tilted its head slightly, as if contemplating her question. Then, in the silence, it mouthed a single word: *"Death."*

Rose's heart stopped. Her mind refused to comprehend what was happening. This wasn't real—this couldn't be real. She closed her eyes tightly, willing the shadow to disappear.

When she opened them, it was gone.

She stood there, breathless, her mind spinning, her body cold with fear. For a moment, she thought it had been a hallucination, a product of stress. But the unease lingered, crawling beneath her skin like a living thing.

She hurried to her bedroom, locking the door behind her. Lying in bed, her heart still pounding, Rose told herself it was nothing. But deep down, she knew the truth—this was just the beginning. The uninvited guest had arrived.

And it wasn't leaving.

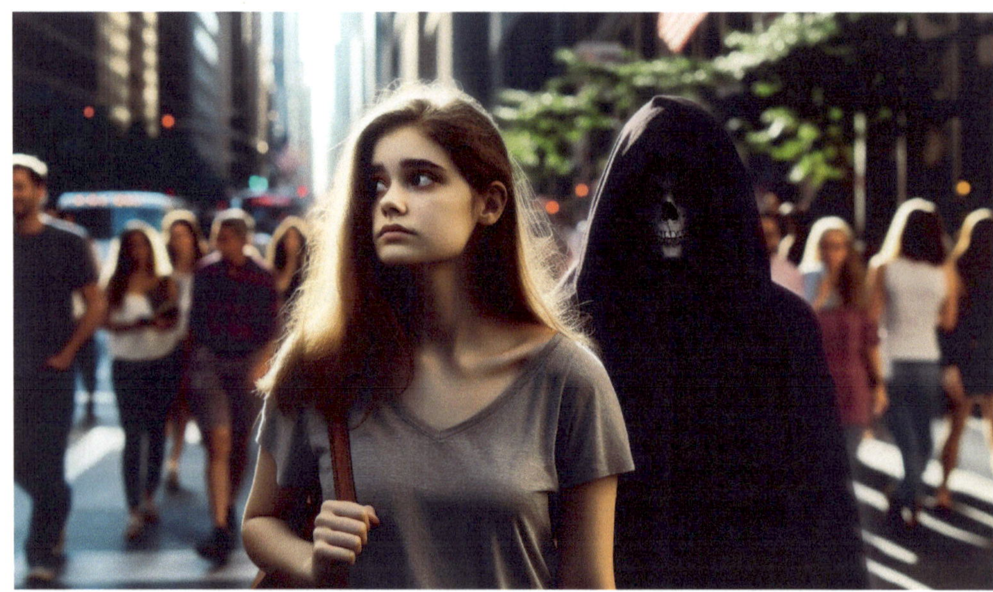

Shadows in the Daylight

The next morning, Rose awoke with a heaviness in her chest. The events of the previous night seemed like a bad dream, but the lingering fear told her it had been all too real. She shook her head, forcing herself to get on with the day.

As she moved through her morning routine, something felt off. It was as if a shadow followed her, just at the edge of her vision. She would catch a glimpse of it in the mirror, a flicker in the corner of the room, but when she turned to face it, nothing was there.

Her anxiety grew. She tried to immerse herself in work, but her concentration wavered. The presence of Death was everywhere—though invisible, its weight was palpable. She canceled plans with friends, preferring the isolation of her apartment. She told herself it was just stress, but the unease gnawed at her.

Days passed, and the presence didn't fade. At times, she could feel it sitting across from her at the dining table, standing behind her as she washed dishes, or lurking in the hallway as she moved from one room to the next. Rose's nerves were frayed, and sleep came only in short, restless spurts. She didn't dare mention it to anyone. After all, who would believe her?

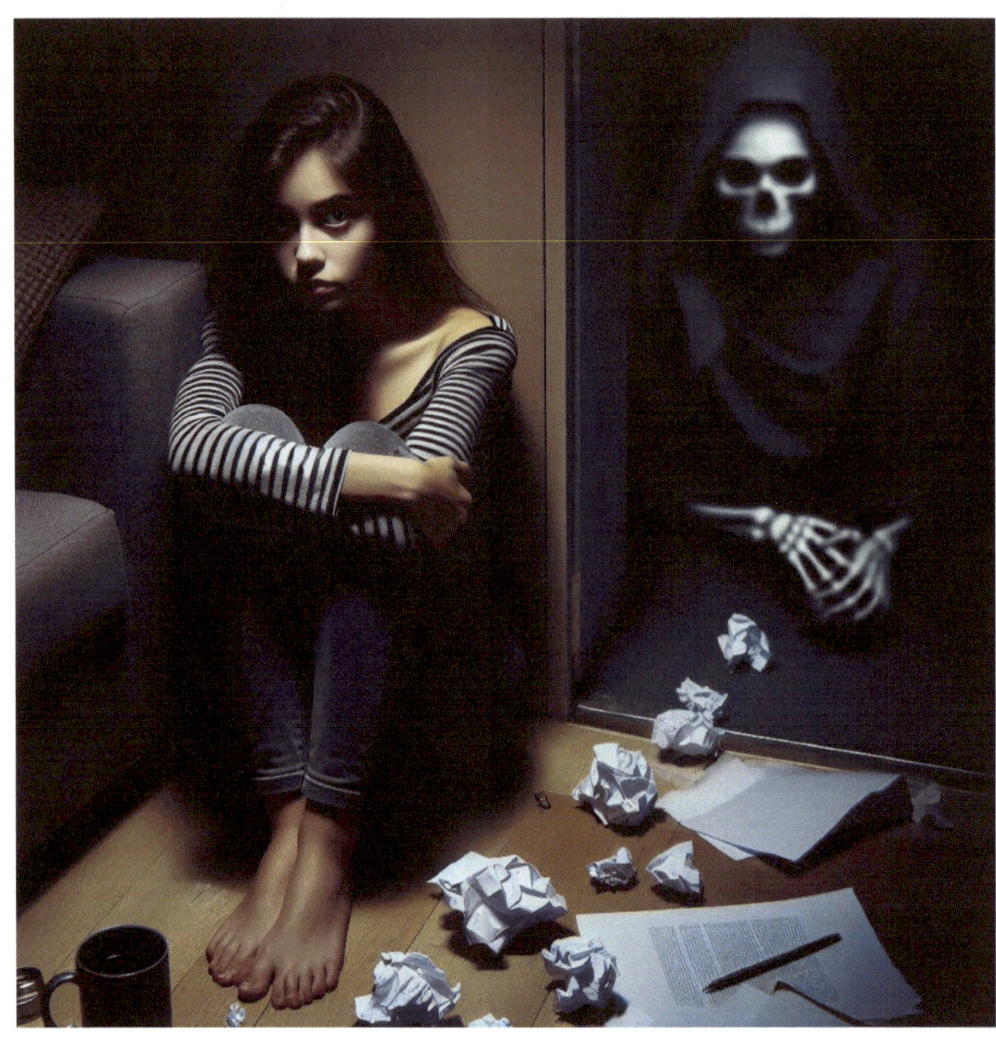

The Spiral Begins

Weeks had gone by, and Rose's world had shrunk to the confines of her apartment. She had stopped going to work, stopped returning calls from friends and family. Her once-vibrant social life had withered, and even the simplest tasks felt insurmountable.

The figure—Death—was now a constant presence, a looming shadow that she could no longer ignore. It never spoke, but its silent company was more terrifying than any words could have been. Every time she tried to leave the apartment, the shadow would appear, blocking the door, as if daring her to step outside.

Rose's mental state deteriorated. She would lie on the couch for hours, staring blankly at the walls, her thoughts clouded with fear and confusion. She tried everything to block it out—music, TV, even alcohol—but nothing worked. The fear had taken root, and her attempts to escape only made it grow stronger.

Friends sent texts and voicemails, but she couldn't bring herself to reply. She didn't want to explain that she was haunted, nor did she want them to see what had become of her. She felt trapped, not just by Death but by her own mind.

She had never felt so alone.

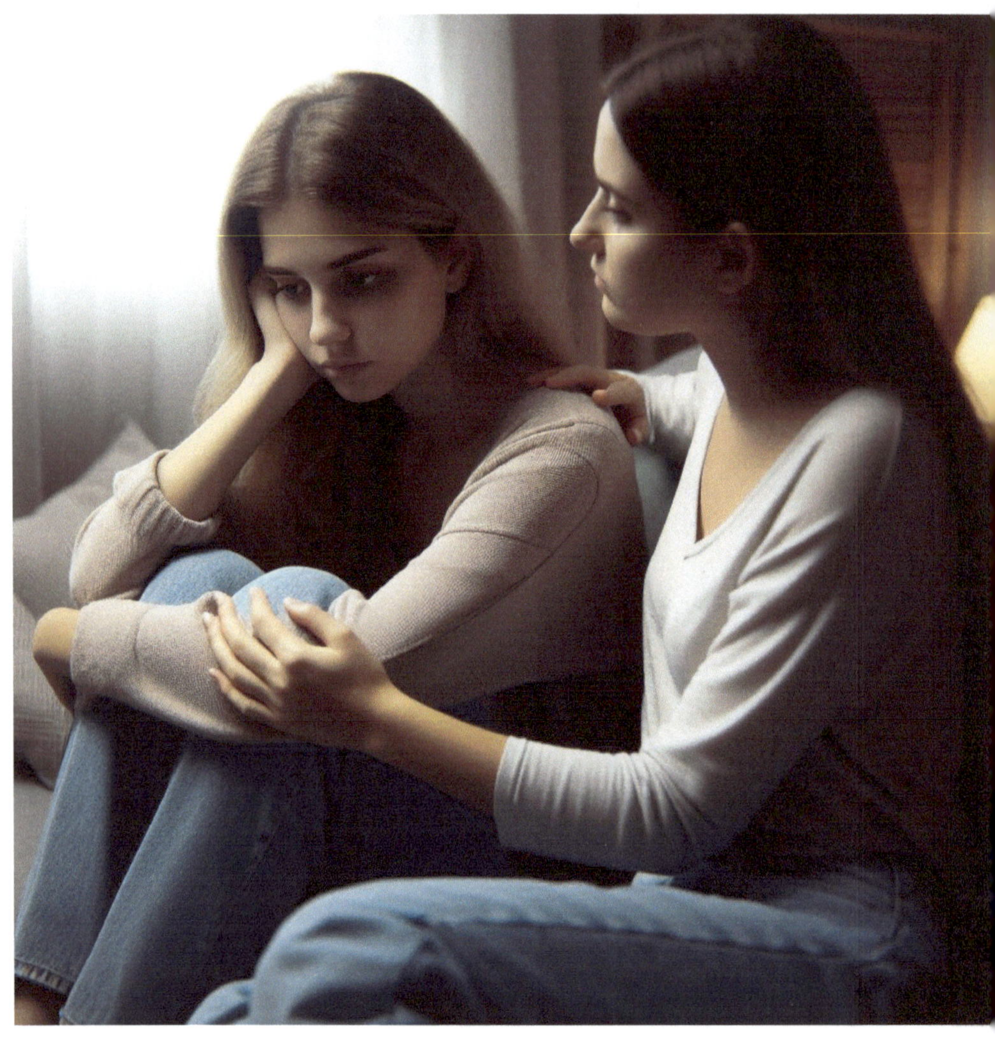

A Friend in Need

It was on a rainy Tuesday afternoon when her phone buzzed yet again. Rose glanced at it with mild irritation, expecting yet another message from a concerned friend. But this time, it was different.

"Rose, I'm worried. Please let me come over. I don't care if you don't want to talk. I just want to see you. Please."

It was a message from Emily, her closest friend, the one person she hadn't entirely shut out. Rose hesitated. She didn't want Emily to see her like this, but something in the message tugged at her. Emily wouldn't give up easily, and deep down, Rose knew she needed someone, anyone, to help her through this.

After what felt like an eternity, Rose replied with a simple, *"Okay."*

When Emily arrived, the tension in the room was thick. Rose hadn't seen anyone for weeks, and the sight of her friend standing at the door, with concern etched on her face, made Rose want to collapse into tears.

But she held herself together.

"Rose, what's going on?" Emily asked gently, stepping inside. Her eyes scanned the apartment, noting the mess, the stale air, and Rose's disheveled appearance. "I've been trying to reach you for days. Why didn't you respond?"

Rose shrugged, looking away. She couldn't bring herself to tell the truth. How could she explain that she was being haunted by something that wasn't real?

"I just... I've been feeling off," she muttered, hoping the conversation would end there.

But Emily wasn't easily convinced. She sat down beside Rose, her voice soft but firm. "This isn't just 'off,' Rose. Something is seriously wrong. You need to talk to someone."

Rose shook her head, her heart racing. "No one can help with this."

Emily's eyes narrowed with concern. "Rose, you're scaring me. Please, let me help."

There was a long silence, the kind that weighed heavily between them. Rose wanted to open up, to spill everything, but the words were trapped in her throat. Finally, after what felt like hours, she whispered, "I think I'm being haunted."

Emily blinked, taken aback by the confession. She waited, giving Rose the space to continue.

"By Death," Rose added quietly, her voice barely above a whisper. "I see it. I feel it. Everywhere I go."

Emily didn't laugh or dismiss her. Instead, she took a deep breath, her expression thoughtful. "I think I know someone who can help."

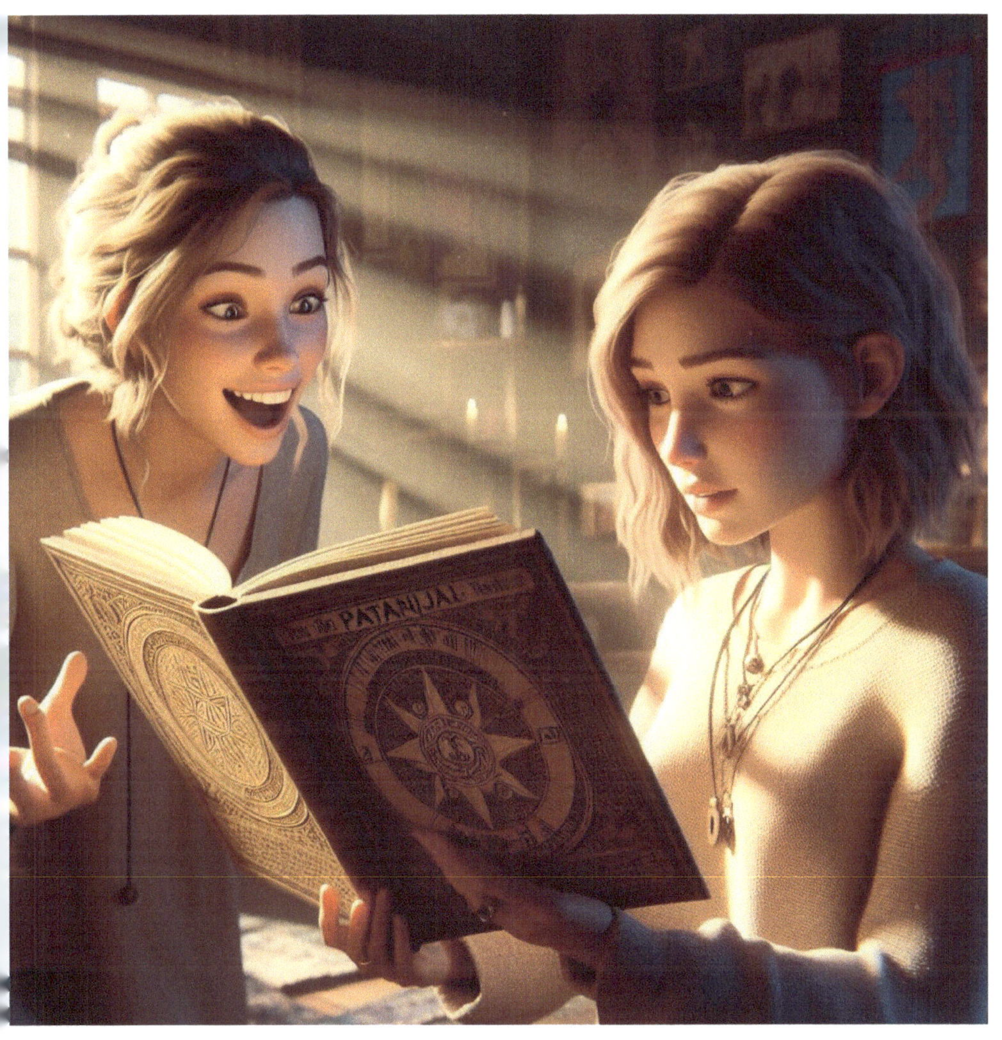

Ancient Wisdom Meets Modern Crisis

Two days later, Emily returned with a book in hand. The cover was worn, the title embossed in gold letters: *The Yoga Sutras of Patanjali*. Rose looked at it with mild skepticism.

"What is this?" she asked.

"It's a guide. An ancient text that teaches how to calm the mind and confront fear," Emily explained. "I've been reading about it. There's something called pranayama—breathing techniques that help bring balance and clarity."

Rose raised an eyebrow. "Breathing is going to help me? Emily, I think I need more than that."

Emily smiled gently. "I know it sounds strange, but hear me out. This isn't just any breathing. It's a practice that's been around for thousands of years. People have used it to overcome fear, anxiety, even existential dread. What if we give it a try?"

Rose hesitated. It all seemed too simple, too... ancient. But at the same time, she had tried everything else, and nothing had worked. Perhaps Emily was right. What did she have to lose?

"Okay," Rose agreed quietly, taking the book from Emily. "I'll try."

Emily's face lit up with relief. "Good. We'll start together. We'll go through the teachings and learn the breathing techniques. And who knows? Maybe this is exactly what you need."

That night, as Rose sat with the ancient book in her hands, she felt a small flicker of hope—a tiny light in the dark, one that she hadn't felt in a long time.

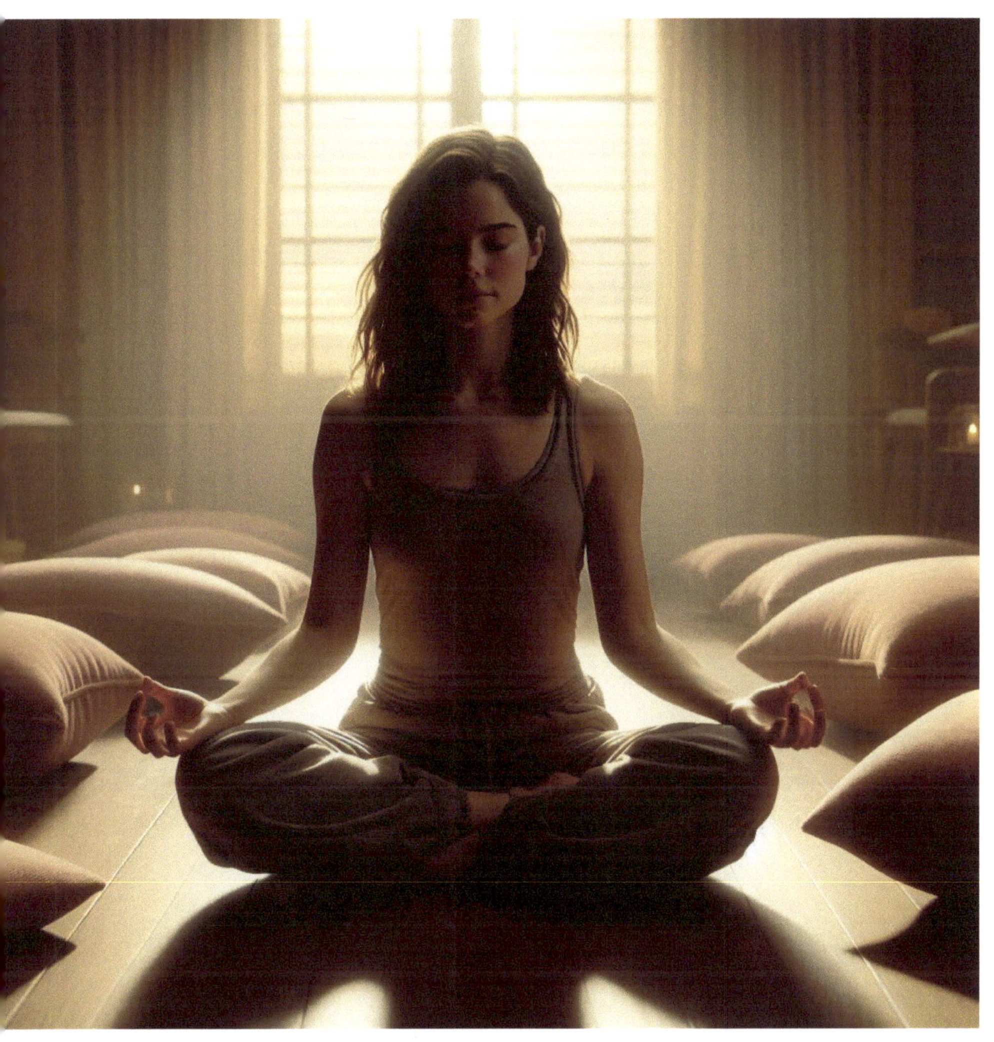

The First Breath

Rose sat cross-legged on the living room floor, facing Emily, who had the book of Patanjali's teachings open on her lap. The air was still, and for the first time in weeks, Rose didn't feel Death's presence looming in the background. But she knew it was still there, waiting in the shadows.

"Okay," Emily said softly. "Let's start simple. Just focus on your breath."

Rose's heart raced. It seemed almost laughable that something so basic could help her, but Emily's steady presence reassured her.

"Close your eyes," Emily instructed. "Inhale slowly and deeply through your nose, and exhale through your mouth. Just let yourself relax."

Rose did as she was told, feeling the air fill her lungs and then leave her body. At first, her breaths were shallow, rushed, like they always were when anxiety struck. But as she focused, the inhales became longer, smoother, and more controlled.

Emily guided her gently through a basic pranayama technique called *Nadi Shodhana*, or alternate nostril breathing. Rose placed one finger on her right nostril, inhaling through the left, then switched sides, exhaling through the right. The rhythm was strange at first, but as she continued, a sense of calm began to creep in.

For the first time in weeks, Rose didn't feel that suffocating tightness in her chest. The shadowy presence of Death, always lurking just out of sight, seemed to shrink, as if it too was affected by the steady rhythm of her breath.

"How do you feel?" Emily asked after a few minutes.

Rose opened her eyes, surprised by the lightness in her body. "Better," she whispered. "Lighter."

Emily smiled. "This is just the beginning. Keep practicing, and you'll see how powerful the breath can be."

Though the fear still lingered, Rose couldn't deny the subtle shift in her perception. The first breath was a small step, but it was a step toward something new.

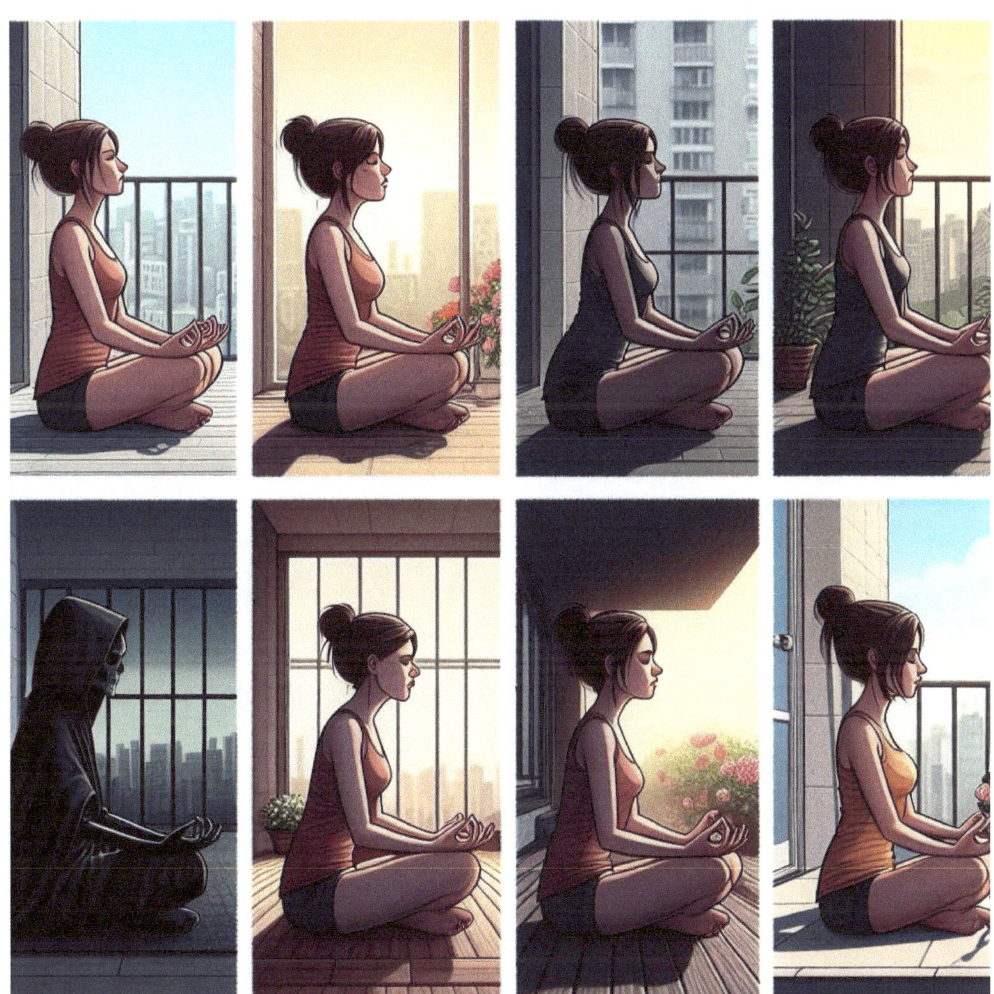

Steady Practice, Unsteady Mind

Days turned into weeks, and Rose began to incorporate pranayama into her daily routine. Each morning, she sat on her bedroom floor, legs crossed, focusing on the steady rise and fall of her breath. At times, the practice felt natural, almost peaceful. Other times, it was a battle.

Death still appeared, especially during the quiet moments when her mind wandered. But now, instead of recoiling in fear, Rose would breathe. She focused on each inhale and exhale, trying to ground herself in the present moment, rather than letting her thoughts spiral.

Despite her growing dedication, there were setbacks. Some days, the anxiety returned with a vengeance. Rose would sit on the floor, gasping for breath, unable to calm the rising panic. On these days, Death felt stronger, closer— its presence overwhelming. But Emily had warned her this would happen.

"Your mind isn't going to let go of fear easily," Emily had said one afternoon. "It's been holding onto it for so long, it doesn't know how to function without it. You just have to be patient with yourself."

Rose tried to heed her friend's advice, but it wasn't easy. The fear that had gripped her for so long was deeply ingrained, and breaking free from it felt impossible at times.

But slowly, incrementally, Rose's mental state began to shift. The panic attacks became less frequent, and when Death did appear, it felt less threatening. It was still there, still looming, but it no longer had the same power over her.

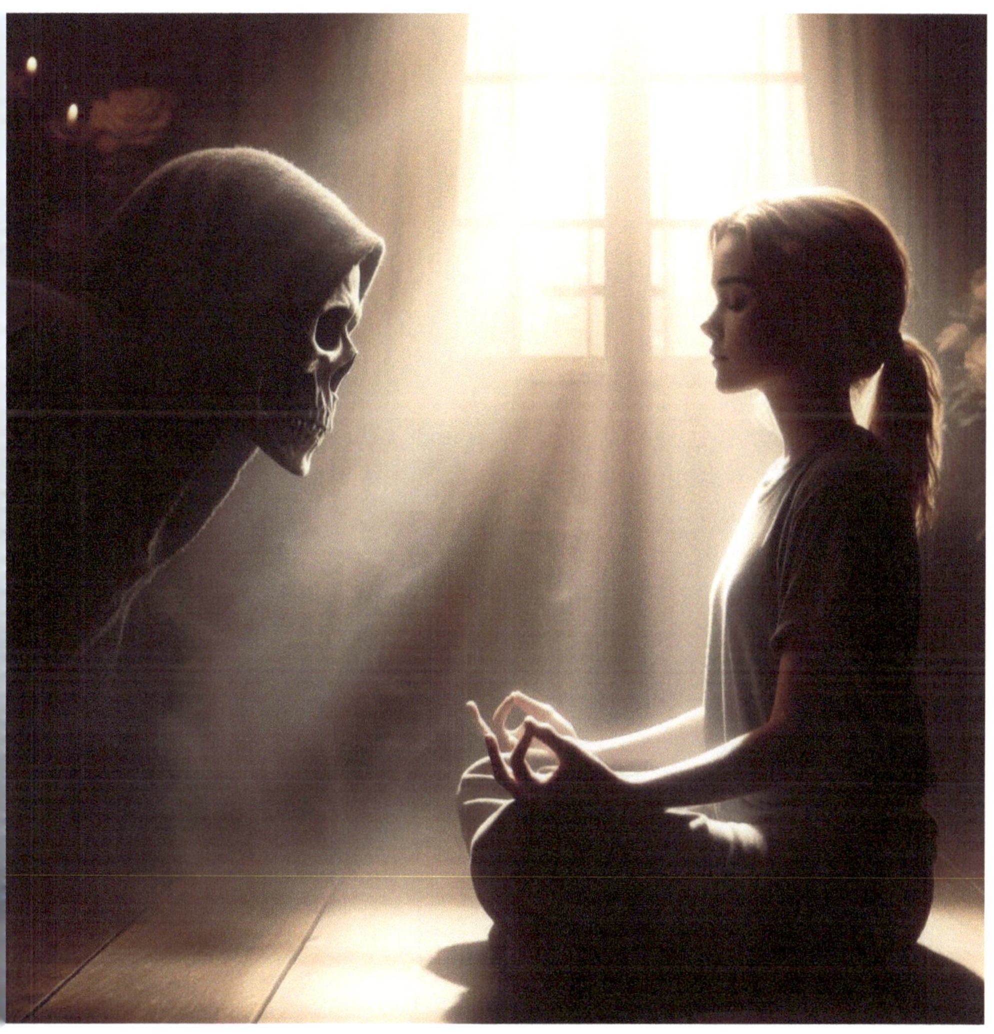

Confronting the Fear

One evening, after an especially exhausting day, Rose sat in her usual spot, focusing on her breath. The apartment was quiet, and she felt herself slipping into a deep meditative state, her mind calm, her body relaxed.

But then, she felt it—the familiar coldness that signaled Death's arrival.

Her eyes flew open, and there it was, standing across the room, its dark form barely visible in the dim light. For a moment, fear gripped her. She wanted to flee, to hide, to do anything but face it.

But this time, Rose didn't run. She didn't turn away. Instead, she closed her eyes and breathed. She focused on the sensation of the air entering and leaving her body, grounding herself in the present moment.

Death moved closer, its presence heavy in the room. Rose's heart raced, but she kept breathing, refusing to give in to the fear.

As Death approached, she felt something shift inside her. The realization hit her like a wave: the more she feared Death, the stronger it became. Her fear was what gave it power, what made it grow. Without that fear, it was just a shadow—a reflection of her own mind.

For the first time, Rose confronted Death not with terror, but with calm. She breathed deeply, her heart steadying, and as she did, Death's form began to blur, its edges dissolving like mist in the morning sun.

It wasn't gone, not yet. But it was fading.

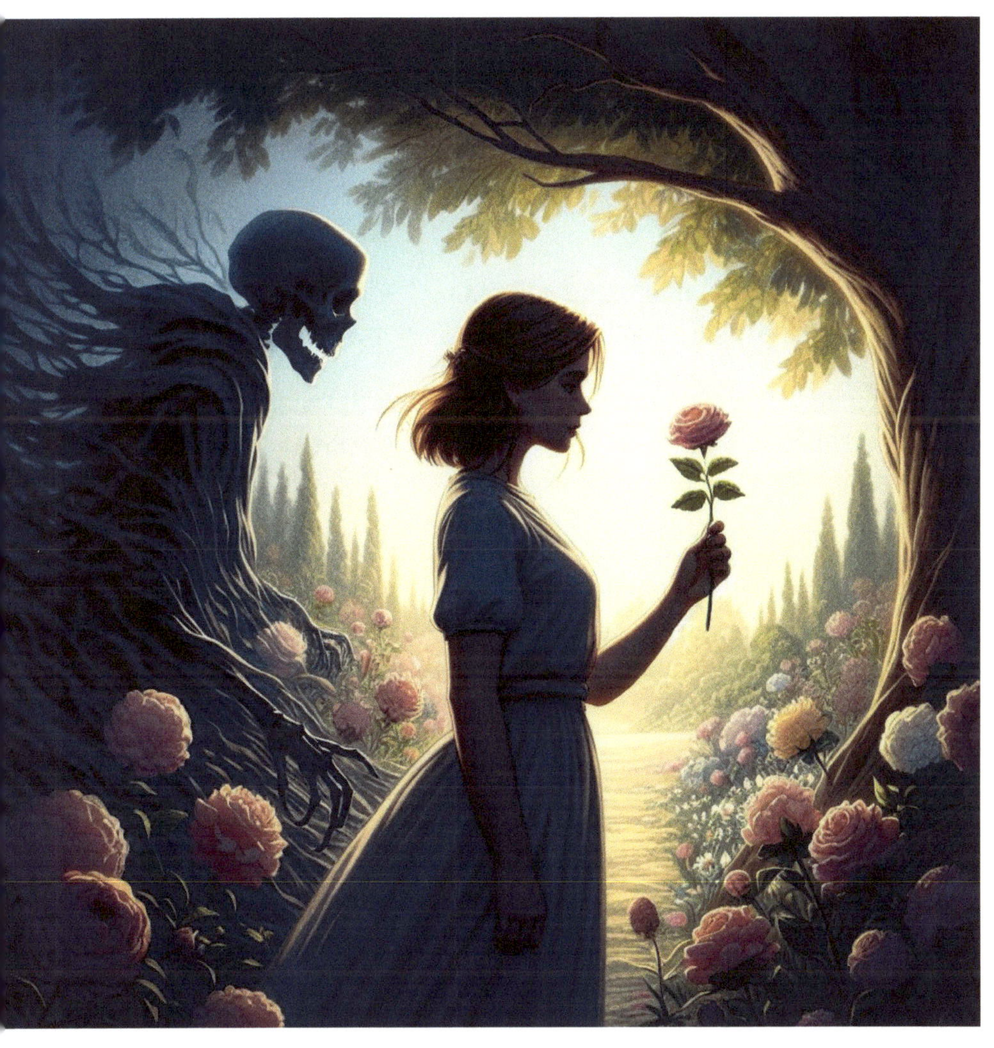

The Nature of Impermanence

The next day, Rose and Emily met at a nearby park, the fresh air a welcome break from the confines of the apartment. They walked in silence for a while, the sound of their footsteps blending with the rustle of leaves.

"I had an experience last night," Rose said finally. "Death came again. But this time... I didn't run."

Emily listened quietly as Rose described the encounter, her face thoughtful. "That's a big step," she said. "You're learning to confront your fear, instead of letting it control you."

"I think I'm starting to understand something," Rose continued. "All of this—life, death, fear—it's all... temporary, isn't it? Nothing stays the same forever."

Emily nodded. "That's one of the core teachings of Patanjali: the concept of impermanence. Everything changes, everything passes. Even fear. Once you realize that, it loses its power over you."

Rose had always struggled with the idea of impermanence. She had clung to the familiar, afraid of the unknown. But now, as she reflected on her recent experiences, she began to see the wisdom in it. Death wasn't something to be feared; it was just another part of life, as temporary and fleeting as anything else.

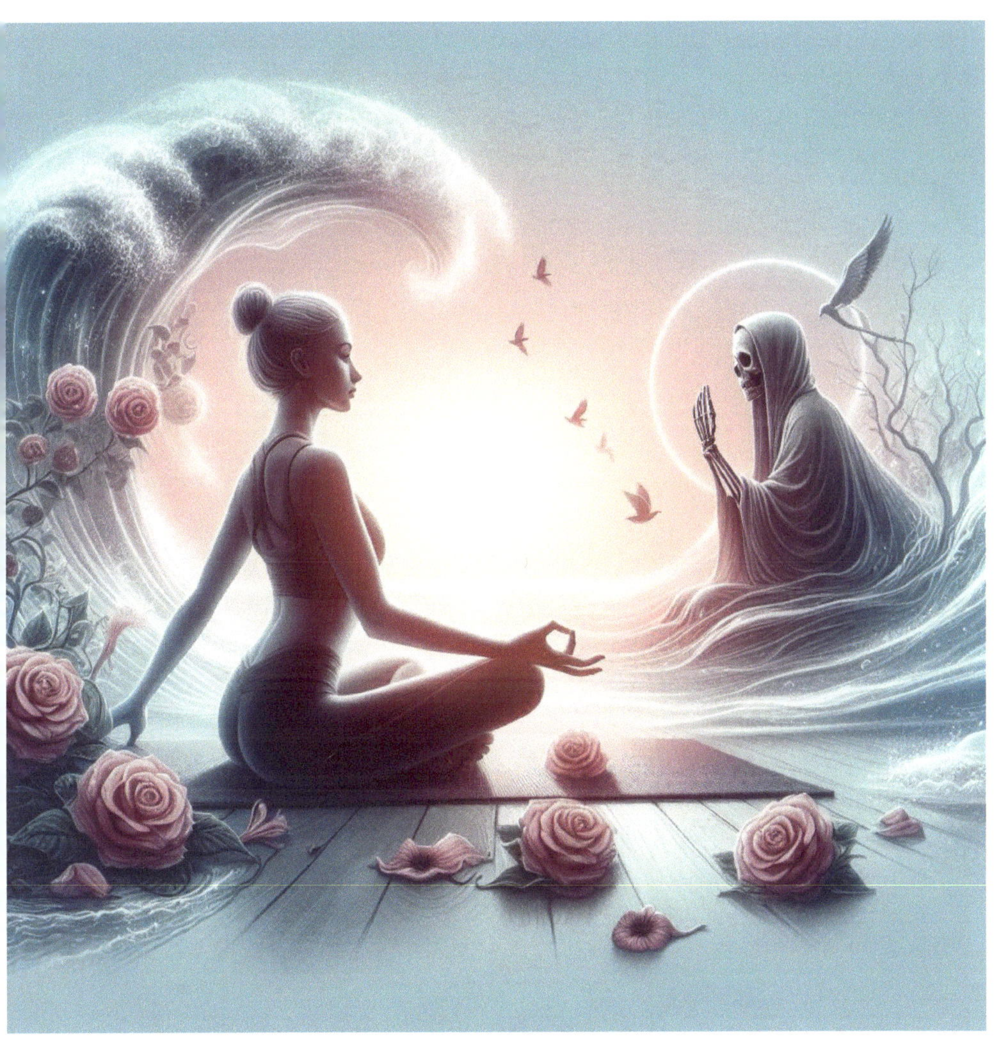

Breath as a Bridge

With a renewed sense of purpose, Rose delved deeper into her pranayama practice. Emily introduced her to more advanced techniques, including *Kapalabhati* (breath of fire) and *Ujjayi* (victorious breath), each designed to bring balance and clarity to the mind.

The breath became more than just a way to calm herself—it became a bridge between her body, mind, and spirit. When fear crept in, she used the breath to ground herself, to center her thoughts. And with each breath, she felt more connected, more at peace.

One morning, after an intense session of pranayama, Rose sat in stillness, her mind clear, her body relaxed. For the first time since Death had appeared, she felt truly at peace. The shadowy presence that had once terrified her was nowhere to be found.

It wasn't that Death had disappeared completely, but rather that its presence no longer consumed her. Through her breath, Rose had found a way to coexist with the fear, without letting it control her.

She was beginning to understand that breath was more than just a tool—it was life itself, a way to connect to something deeper, something eternal.

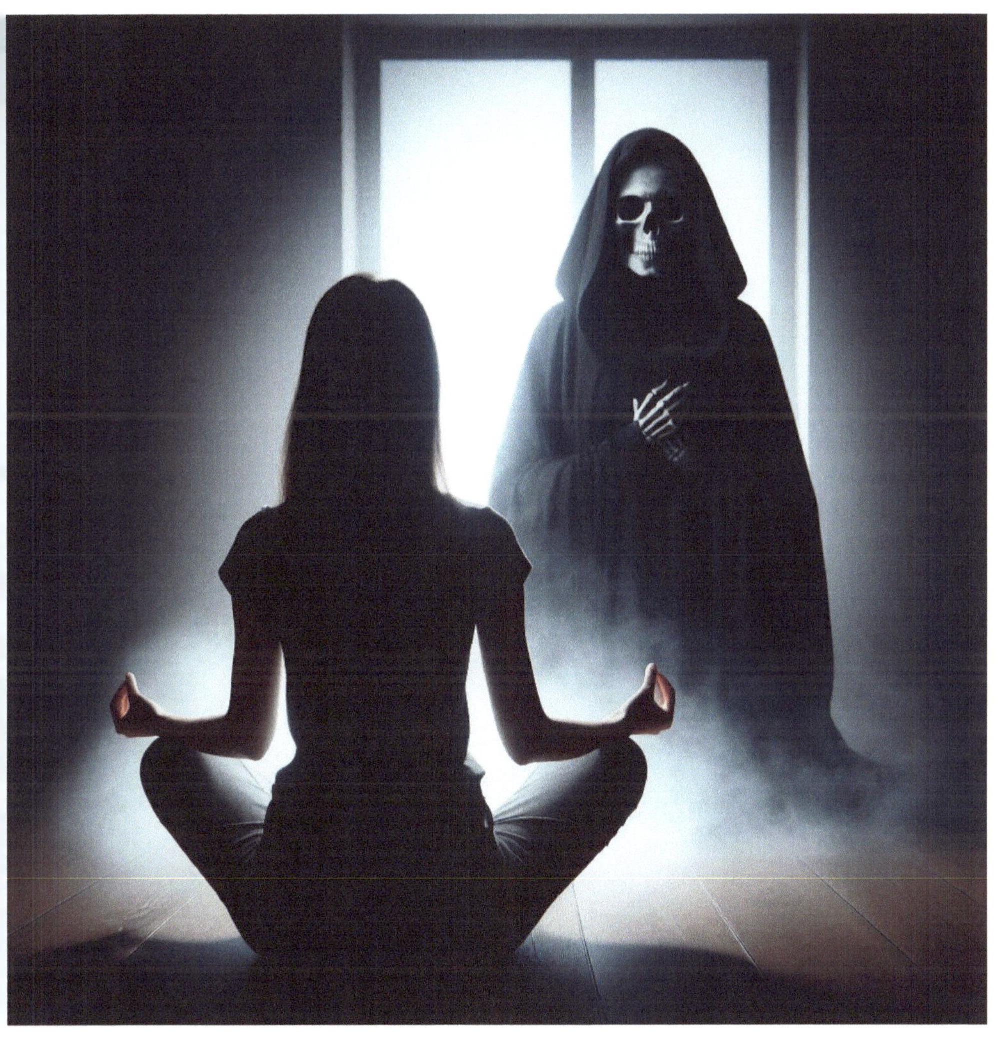

Death as a Teacher

It had been weeks since Rose began her steady pranayama practice, and something profound had shifted within her. She no longer dreaded the shadow of Death that sometimes appeared in her apartment or followed her in her dreams. In fact, Rose now greeted its presence with a strange sense of calm, even curiosity.

Death was no longer just a terrifying figure that loomed in the background of her life. It had become something else entirely—a teacher.

One evening, as she sat on the floor in meditation, Death appeared again, this time closer than it had ever been before. But instead of recoiling, Rose remained still, her breath even and controlled. She opened her eyes and looked at it—not with fear, but with understanding.

"You're not here to take me, are you?" Rose said quietly, her voice steady.

The shadow did not answer, but its presence felt different—less menacing, more neutral. Rose realized then that Death had never been a threat. It was simply a reminder, a reflection of her own unresolved fears.

"You've been teaching me all along," Rose whispered, as though speaking to an old friend.

Death's presence, once suffocating, now felt like an opportunity. It was showing her something deeper about life itself—that life's beauty and value are only fully appreciated when one confronts its inevitable end. Death was not a punishment or a terror to be avoided, but a guide, pointing her toward a deeper understanding of existence.

Rose smiled faintly, feeling a surge of gratitude. She closed her eyes again and focused on her breath, letting the presence of Death blend into the background.

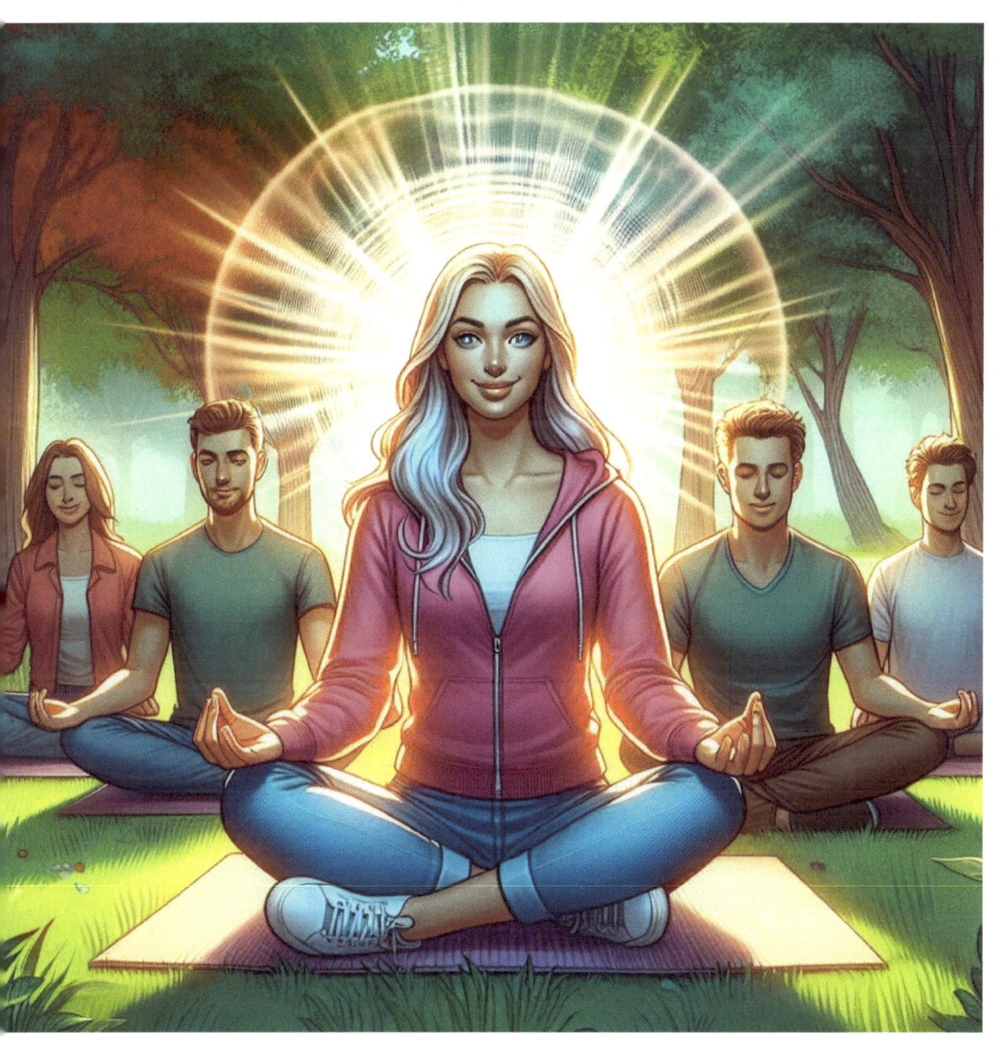

The Ripple Effect

The changes in Rose's life were becoming visible to everyone around her. She had started going out again—meeting friends for coffee, reconnecting with family, even going back to work part-time. There was a lightness in her that hadn't been there before, a sense of calm that radiated in her presence.

Emily noticed it most. One evening, as they sat together on Rose's couch, Emily smiled and said, "You're like a completely different person."

Rose laughed softly. "I don't know if I'm different. Maybe I just finally understand something I didn't before."

She had begun sharing bits and pieces of her journey with her friends. At first, she was hesitant, unsure if they would understand her experience with Death or the teachings of Patanjali. But as she spoke about her fears and the transformative power of pranayama, she found that people were more open than she had expected. Some even asked her to teach them the breathing techniques.

"I think I might start a small group," Rose said one afternoon. "You know, to teach pranayama and share what I've learned. There are so many people who struggle with fear and anxiety. Maybe this could help them too."

Emily beamed with pride. "That's a wonderful idea, Rose. You've come so far. I think people could really benefit from your experience."

And so, the ripple effect began. Rose started with a few friends, guiding them through basic breathing exercises and sharing the wisdom she had gained from her own journey. Slowly but surely, her small group grew, and with each person she helped, Rose felt more and more connected to her purpose.

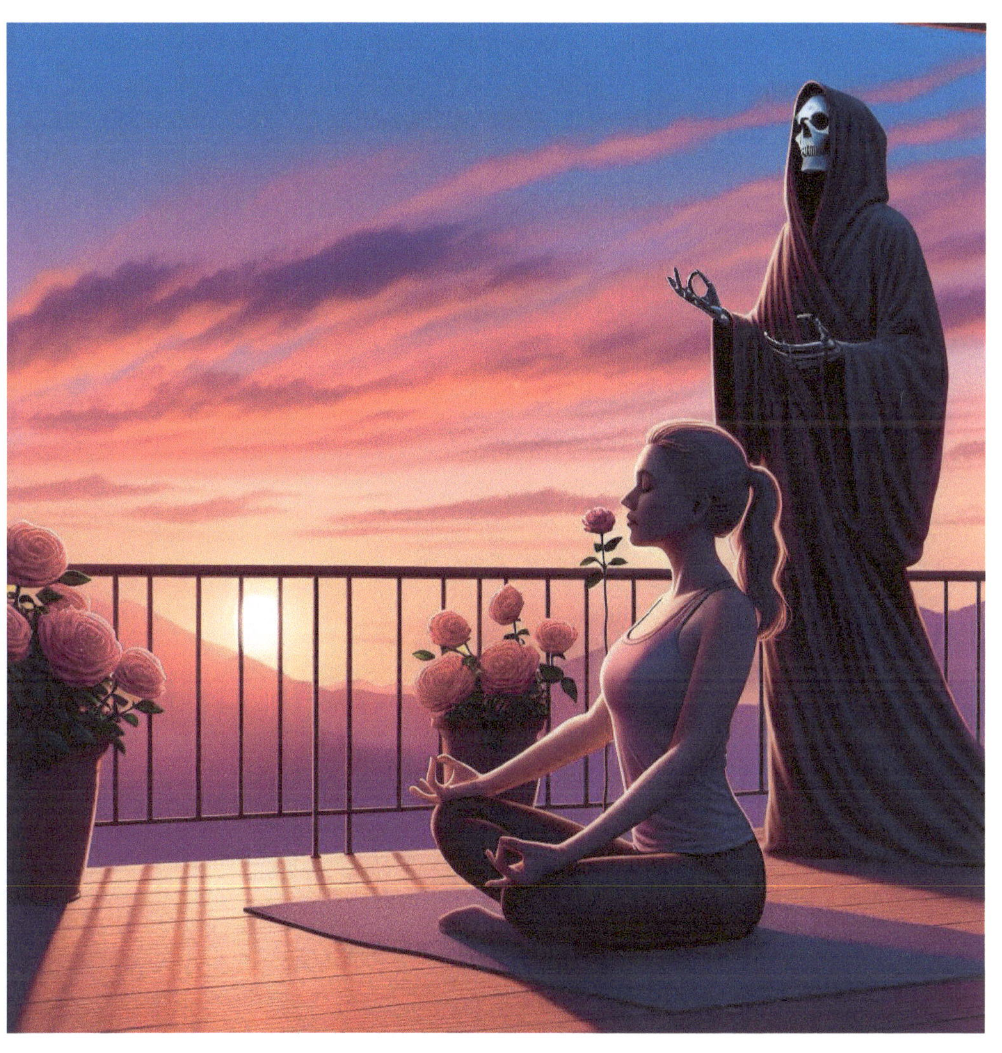

Dancing with the Shadows

Rose's relationship with Death had transformed from one of terror to one of acceptance. She no longer feared the shadowy figure that once haunted her, but instead, she learned to dance with it.

Death still appeared from time to time, especially during moments of stress or uncertainty. But instead of freezing in fear, Rose welcomed its presence, using the opportunity to center herself, to breathe deeply and return to her inner calm. She saw Death not as an enemy, but as a reminder that life was precious, and that every breath was a gift.

One evening, after a particularly challenging day, Rose sat on her balcony, watching the sunset. She felt a familiar chill—the presence of Death at her side. Instead of panicking, she closed her eyes and smiled.

"Hello again," she whispered.

She began to practice *Kapalabhati*, the breath of fire, feeling the rush of energy as her body responded. The rhythm of her breath steadied her, and with each exhale, she felt the weight of the day lift off her shoulders.

Death, ever-present but no longer frightening, seemed to linger only to observe. Rose felt a strange sense of companionship, as though Death was merely there to remind her of the fragility of life—not to haunt her, but to guide her toward appreciating every moment.

As the sun dipped below the horizon, Rose opened her eyes, feeling a deep sense of peace. She had learned to dance with her fear, to face it head-on, and in doing so, she had taken control of her own life.

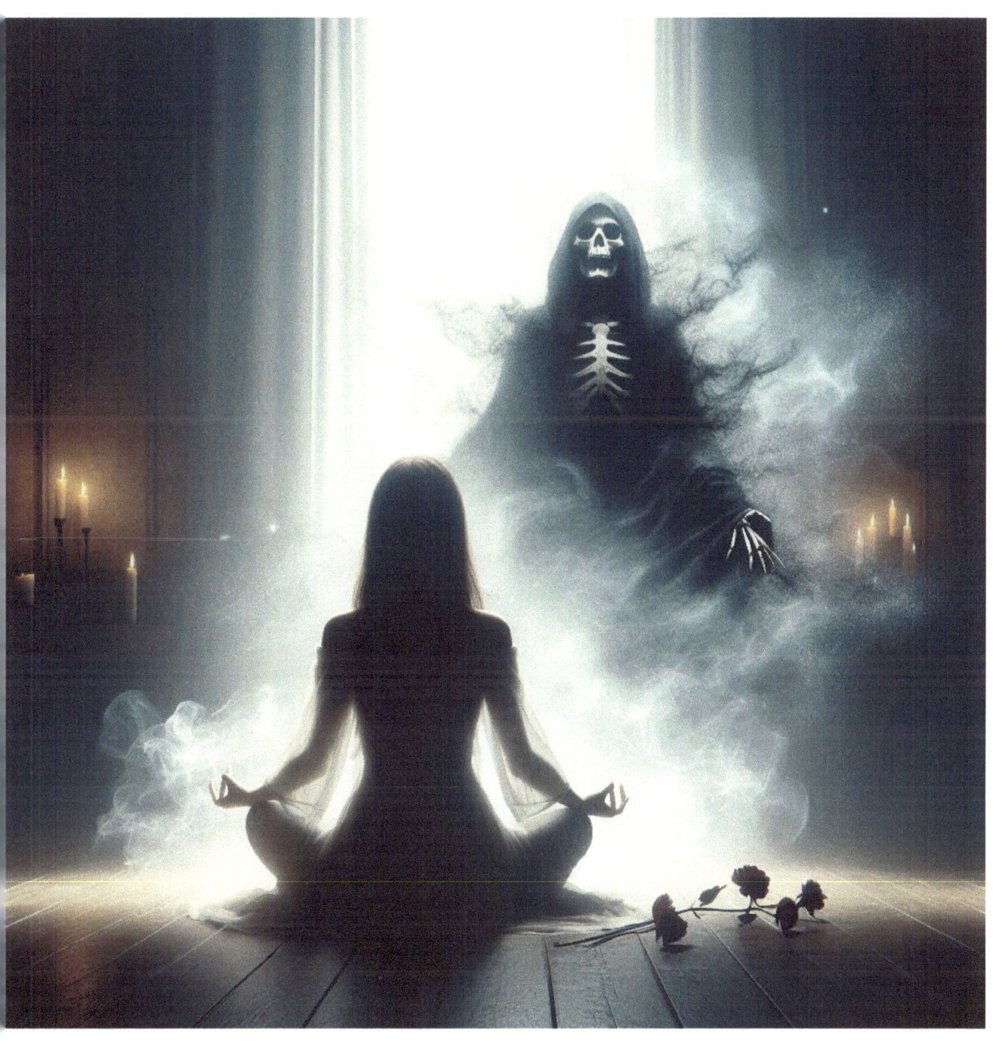

The Uninvited Guest Departs

One evening, as Rose sat in her usual spot, breathing deeply in meditation, she felt something shift. The presence of Death appeared again, as it had many times before. But this time, something was different.

There was no fear, no tension in the air. Instead, Rose felt only a profound sense of peace, as if she had finally completed a long and difficult journey.

She opened her eyes and saw Death standing across the room, its shadowy form as still as ever. But instead of the familiar weight of dread, Rose felt only gratitude.

"Thank you," she said softly, her voice filled with sincerity.

In that moment, she realized that Death had never been a real, external force. It had been a projection of her own inner fears, her own anxieties about the unknown. And now, as she faced it with acceptance, it began to dissolve, fading into the air like mist.

Rose smiled as the room grew lighter. Death, the uninvited guest that had once dominated her life, was gone. It had never been an enemy—only a reflection of the fear she had carried within herself.

With a deep, steady breath, Rose felt an overwhelming sense of liberation. She had confronted her deepest fear, and in doing so, she had freed herself.

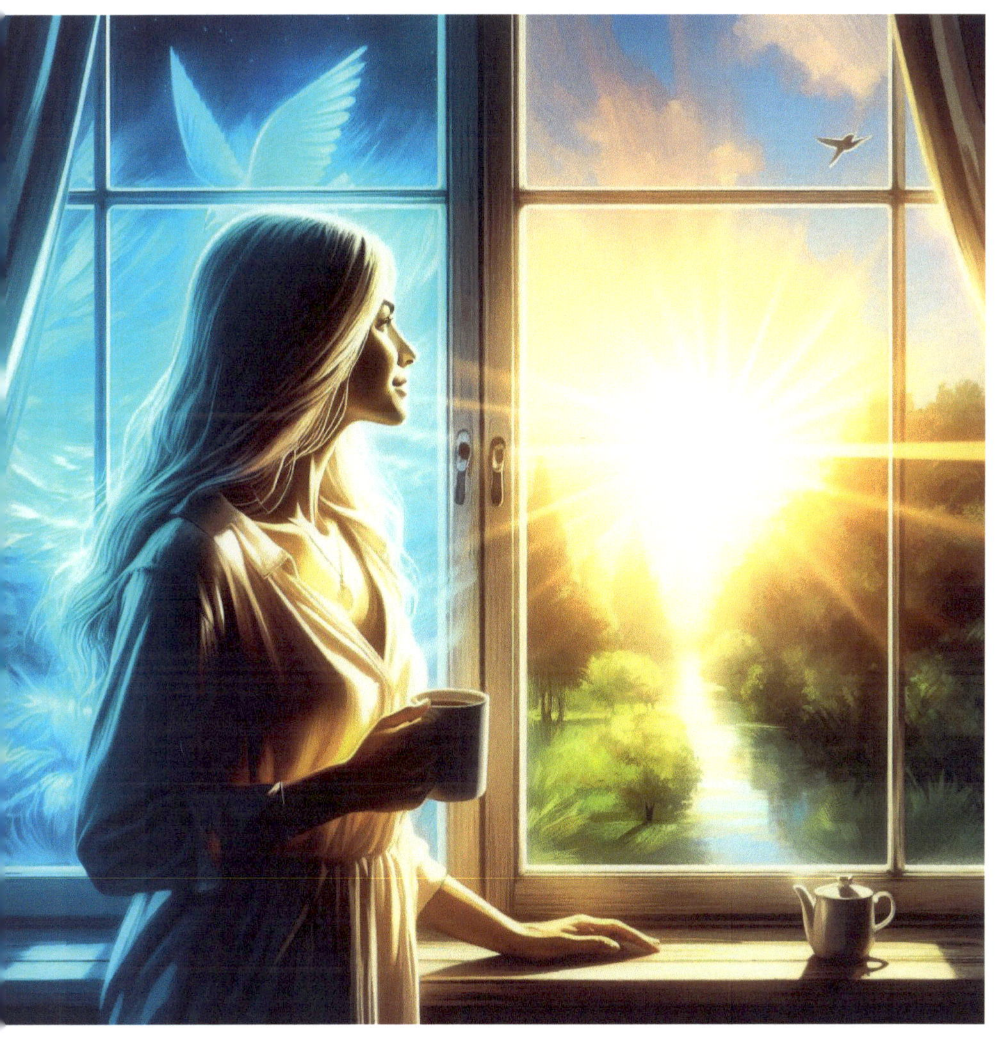

A New Dawn

The next morning, Rose woke with a clarity she hadn't felt in years. The sun streamed through her window, filling the room with warmth and light. She stretched, breathing in the fresh air, and felt an immense sense of peace.

Her journey wasn't over. In fact, she knew it was just beginning. She continued her pranayama practice every day, not because she was afraid, but because it had become an essential part of who she was. The breath had become her anchor, a way to connect with the world, with herself, and with the deeper truths of life.

As she sipped her morning tea, Rose reflected on the path she had traveled. She had faced her fears, learned to breathe through the darkness, and emerged stronger and more grounded than ever before.

The world outside her window seemed brighter, more alive. The fear of Death no longer hung over her like a storm cloud. Instead, she saw life in all its beauty and fragility, and she embraced it fully.

She had found peace—not in avoiding Death, but in understanding it, in seeing it as part of the great cycle of existence. And with that understanding, Rose was ready to live her life fully, without fear.